LOW BACK PAIN
SOLUTIONS SO THAT IT DOES NOT LIMIT YOUR LIFE

JELEEL TEMITOPE RAHEEM

ISBN: 9798390184608

DEDICATION

This is dedicated to my grandpa and all those elders out there

CONTENTS

1   INTRODUCTION

2   What is low back pain?

3   **Types and causes of low back pain**

4   **symptoms of low back pain**

5   **Diagnosis of low back pain**

6   **Treatment of low back pain**

7   **Recommendations for low back pain**

INTRODUCTION

Eight out of ten people have suffered an episode of low back pain at some time in their lives. If you suffer from dorsal pain, find out what type of low back pain affects you and how you can remedy it.

What is low back pain?

Low back pain is defined as pain, from any cause, in the area of the back, from the last ribs to the gluteal folds. Low back pain is very common, Eight out of 10 people experience at least one episode in their lives.

It is the leading cause of disability for people between the ages of 19 and 45, and the second most common cause of lost work days due to disability in adults under 45 (after the common cold).

Low back pain becomes more common as you get older. It affects half of all people over the age of 60 at some point. Its economic impact is considerable. Thus, although low back pain is rarely caused by life-threatening diseases, it is an important health problem. However, the number of back injuries originating in the workplace is declining, perhaps because there is greater awareness of the problem and preventive measures have improved.

The spinal column is made up of the back bones (vertebrae), which are separated and protected by cartilage discs that absorb shocks. The vertebrae are also covered in a thin layer of cartilage and are held in place by ligaments and muscles that help stabilize the spine. The spinal cord is surrounded by the vertebral column. Throughout the entire spinal cord, spinal nerves exit through the spaces between the vertebrae and connect with other nerves throughout the body. The part of the spinal nerve closest to the spinal cord is called the spinal nerve root. Due to their position, the spinal nerve roots can be compressed when the vertebral column is injured, which causes pain.

The lower (lumbar) part of the spine consists of five vertebrae. Connects the chest to the pelvis and legs, providing mobility to twist, bend, and stoop, as well as strength to stand, walk, and lift. Thus, the lumbar region is involved in almost all daily activities. Low back pain limits or prevents these activities and alters the quality of life.

Types and causes of low back pain

We could divide the types of low back pain into two large groups depending on the cause that originates it:

Specific low back pain

That is when the cause is known, which happens only in 20% of cases. In 5% of patients, low back pain is a symptom of a serious underlying disease. These are the causes that should be ruled out in the emergency department.

In 15% of cases, it is a specific alteration of the non-serious area.

Below are different examples of causes of low back pain, which are specific diseases with a specific treatments:

- **Osteoarthritis (degenerative arthritis)** causes a deterioration of the cartilage that covers and protects the vertebrae. This disorder is believed to be due in part to wear and tear from years of use. The discs located between the vertebrae deteriorate, narrowing the spaces and compressing the spinal nerve roots, and irregular bony projections sometimes develop on the vertebrae, which also compress the spinal nerve roots. All of these changes can cause lower back pain and stiffness.
- In **osteoporosis**, bone density decreases, making the bones more brittle (more prone to fracture). The vertebrae in particular are susceptible to the effects of osteoporosis, often causing crush (compression) fractures, which can lead to sudden, severe back pain, and compression of the spinal nerve roots (which can cause back pain). chronic back). However, most fractures due to osteoporosis occur in the upper and mid back and cause pain in those areas rather than in the lower back.
- **Herniated or ruptured or herniated disc**. Each disk has a resistant cover and its interior is soft and gelatinous. If a disc is suddenly compressed by the vertebrae above and below it, the covering can tear (rupture), causing pain. The inside of the disc can break through the tear in the cover so that part of the inside bulges out (herniates). This bulge can compress, irritate, and even injure the spinal nerve root next to it, causing more pain.
- **Spinal stenosis** (narrowing of the spinal canal, which runs through the center of the spine and contains the spinal cord). Spinal stenosis, which in the elderly is a common cause of low back pain, can occur in middle-aged people who have a narrow spinal canal from birth.

In some systemic diseases with an immunological profile such as ankylosing spondylitis, there may be a specific inflammatory affectation of the lower back with decreased flexibility over time. Others, such as psoriasis, the inflammatory disease (

Crohn's disease), can cause secondary involvement of this area of the spine with a significant decrease in the quality of life of the affected person. In the same way, some tumors that settle in structures close to this anatomical zone (kidneys, pancreas) or metastases in the vertebrae of tumors of other organs can cause low back pain.

Referred pain (originating in other organs or parts of the body) tends to be deep, achy, constant, and relatively widespread (diffuse). It is characteristically unaffected by movement and is worse at night. It can originate in another part of the body, such as the kidneys, bladder, uterus, or prostate, but is felt in the lower back.

Nonspecific low back pain

It constitutes the remaining 80%. In these cases, it is not possible to identify the structure that causes the pain. It is a benign process of limited duration, although recurrent, more frequent in middle-aged adults and women. The factors that most frequently can trigger the first episode are: picking up loads, adopting incorrect postures, vibrations, a low level of job satisfaction, obesity, pregnancy, psychological factors, and stress.

From a practical point of view, low back pain can be classified as acute (less than 7 days of evolution), subacute (between 7 days and 7 weeks), and chronic (more than 7 weeks).

In addition, we must take into account other very frequent diseases that can cause low back pain.

The main symptom of low back pain is localized pain in the area between the last ribs and the iliac crests. In most cases, especially in those of unspecific cause, the description of the pain is vague, considering pain on both sides of the spine.

On other occasions, it can refer to a specific area, and can then mean a problem with a specific cause. In most of these cases, they are usually due to contractures of the muscles adjacent to the spine simply due to poor postural hygiene. Unilateral or specific pain on one side is also present with trauma. In these situations, the pain has mechanical characteristics, understood as pain that worsens with activity and is largely relieved with rest and rest.

In other more specific cases, such as low back pain due to disc problems, whether they are herniated or protrusive, the lumbar pain radiates or follows a route that is that of the inflamed nerve root due to the irritation of the damaged disc. The most typical case is sciatica, following a route through the back of the thigh that can reach the foot. Depending on the degree of involvement, sensitivity may be affected, noticing tingling or numbness in some areas of the leg, or strength, manifesting as an inability to walk or lift the limb. The pain of a vertebral fracture due to an osteoporotic process is usually very acute and disabling, requiring a powerful analgesic treatment.

In low back pain due to systemic diseases such as ankylosing spondylitis, the pain is not mechanical, but inflammatory, and this means that rest worsens the symptoms, pain, and functional impotence being more pronounced in the mornings after a night's rest.

Diagnosis of low back pain

When diagnosing low back pain, the main objective when evaluating the patient is to rule out those serious causes whose clinical manifestation is low back pain and which, although infrequent, may require immediate treatment (trauma, infections, tumors...). For this, a clinical history and physical examination will be carried out, paying special attention to the presence of risk factors that make us suspect a serious origin of the pain, which are:

Age over 55 years.

Previous diagnosis of cancer.

Previous diagnosis of severe systemic disease.

History of spinal trauma.

History of recent surgery (spinal or not).

Chronic pulmonary, urinary, or skin infection.

Injecting drug use.

History of immunosuppression (transplant, HIV, etc.).

Prolonged treatment with glucocorticoids.

Duration of pain greater than a month.

Absence of relief with bed rest.

Recent onset of urinary or fecal incontinence.

Exploratory findings:

Unexplained fever.

Unexplained striking weight loss.

Abdominal mass.

Neurological alterations such as loss of strength in the lower limbs, urinary or fecal incontinence…

Depending on the presence or absence of these warning signs, the patient can be classified as:

Patient with suspected specific pathology

The study should be started with a simple radiograph and an analytical one. Depending on the results and clinical suspicion, other diagnostic tests will be performed. Regarding imaging tests, depending on the suspicion, X-rays, CT scans, magnetic resonance imaging or other more specific ones will be performed.

Patient with non-specific low back pain

Although the data available to establish guidelines for clinical action are incomplete, due to the scarcity of well-designed studies, in the absence of suspicion of a serious etiology of the pain, laboratory studies are not recommended (complete blood count, sedimentation rate, biochemistry, and laboratory tests). urine), imaging tests (x-ray, resonance, or CT), or other diagnostic techniques during the first month of evolution, even in patients with clinical suspicion of disc herniation.

Most people with back pain will improve within a month, with or without treatment, so the initial management of a patient with acute low back pain without associated risk factors should be conservative, to achieve symptomatic relief. If there is no improvement with adequate treatment in that period, the case should be reconsidered and the appropriate complementary tests performed

Treatment of low back pain

Depending on the type of pain suffered, the treatment of low back pain will be one way or another:

Low back pain secondary to the severe or specific pathology

The cause must be treated, with the specific treatment for it.

Nonspecific acute low back pain

The main measure during the acute phase has traditionally been absolute bed rest; however, studies have shown that bed rest of more than two days is more detrimental in terms of pain and functional disability than an active attitude, so it is recommended to resume walking and usual activities as soon as possible (except for heavy physical labor). Postural re-education aimed at avoiding activities and postures that trigger pain is advisable.

Pharmacological treatment is based on analgesic drugs (paracetamol), anti-inflammatories, and muscle relaxants (the latter, no more than two weeks).

Starting from the second week, light aerobic exercise should be recommended, and, from the fourth week, flexibility and trunk strengthening exercises.

If the symptoms persist for more than 4-6 weeks despite conservative treatment or the intensity increases during it, it is necessary to reassess the patient completely, performing diagnostic tests and specific treatments, if necessary.

Recurrent nonspecific acute low back pain

The acute episode should be treated as indicated. There is moderate evidence in favor of the use of aerobic physical exercise, flexibility, and trunk strengthening as long-term prevention to reduce episodes of acute low back pain.

Nonspecific subacute low back pain

Once the treatment of the acute phase is completed, it is recommended not to leave analgesic treatment for longer than necessary. Exercise combined with behavioral therapy (taking care of postures above all) has shown moderate efficacy in these cases.

Nonspecific chronic low back pain

When the pain persists for more than 12 weeks (three months), the diagnosis of chronic low back pain is established. In these cases, if the physical examination allows ruling out serious pathology, no diagnostic method is recommended unless a specific cause is suspected.

The treatment aims to ensure that the patient has normal physical activity. Exercise programs and behavioral therapies have proven useful; however, physical therapy (heat or cold, brace, laser, ultrasound) is not recommended in these patients. For pain, analgesia should be prescribed at short intervals of time; antidepressants and muscle relaxants can help control this symptom.

Interventional measures, such as acupuncture or epidural or intra-articular corticosteroids, have not been effective. In certain cases, the possibility of referring the patient to pain units should be considered for long-term treatment.

Surgery may be an option for cases of chronic low back pain of more than two years in which all conservative measures have failed and there is degenerative disc disease of one or two levels.

In the management of these patients, the prevention of disability due to low back pain is also essential, for which the following strategies are useful: placing equal emphasis on relieving pain as on recovering function, recommending that patients continue to be active, diverting resources to active treatment modalities (avoid massages, passive rehabilitation, prolonged rest, acupuncture, etc., since there is no evidence of their efficacy)

Recommendations for low back pain

If you suffer from low back pain, the following tips will help you cope and ease the pain:

Exercise regularly and adapted to the individual's capacity.

Two types of exercises can be helpful: aerobic exercises (such as swimming) and stretching and strengthening exercises for specific muscles (such as pelvic tilts and abdominal flexions). Some techniques such as those used in Pilates can favor the lumbar muscles and prevent injuries.

Avoid standing or sitting for prolonged periods, as well as postures or movements that cause pain. It is advisable when you have to stand for a long period to rest on one of the legs, avoiding standing on both at the same time.

Maintain good posture when the person is standing or sitting. In the chair, the 90º position marked by the chair itself must be ensured, in such a way that this angle is formed between the thighs and the back.

Sleep in a comfortable position on a firm mattress. When adopting the lateral position in bed, it is advisable to place a small cushion or pillow between the legs so that the two knees do not come into contact. In the same way, when getting out of bed, it should be done in lateral decubitus, lowering the legs first to later separate the trunk from the mattress utilizing the arm.

Some postural exercises at home can alleviate this problem, especially those in which the back rests on the floor and the legs are flexed with the help of the arms towards the abdomen, or placing the legs on the seat of a chair forming 90º between the thighs and the trunk.

Learn to lift objects correctly (bend the knees sufficiently so that the arms are at the level of the object to be lifted).

CONCLUSION

I hope and believed that I have helped you in solving and finding a lasting solution to the Low back pain and I wish you follow the layout there and get better always.

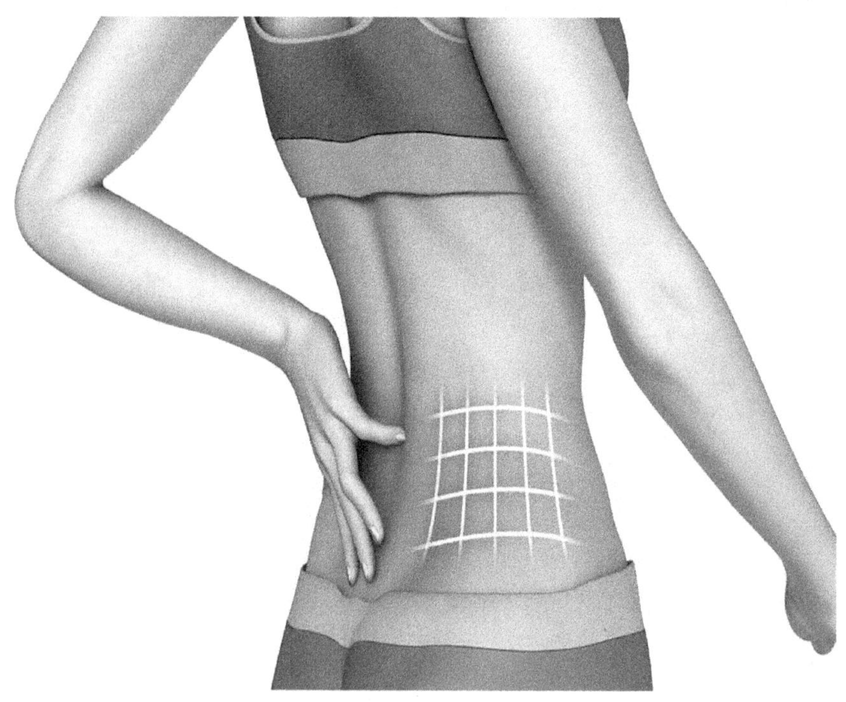

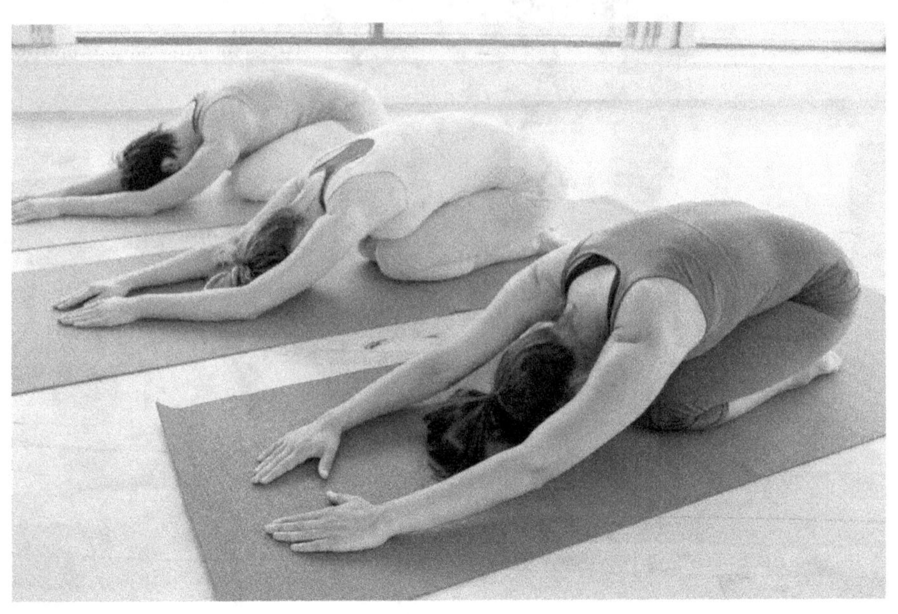

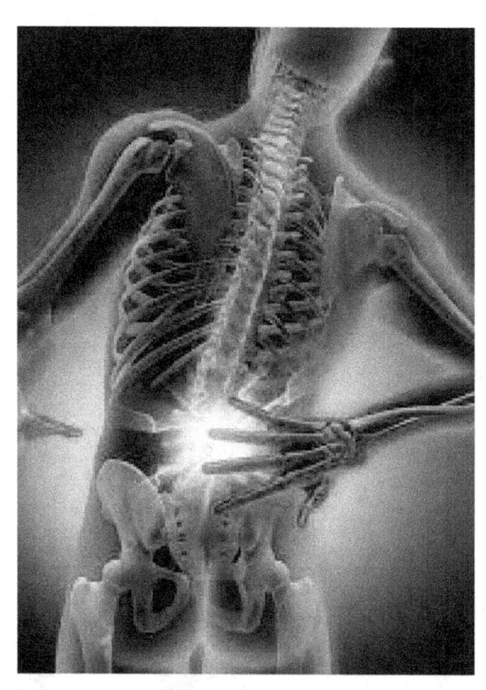

ABOUT THE AUTHOR

JELEEL TEMITOPE RAHEEM is a good trainer and also a certified Chemist who loves researching for better health of the people

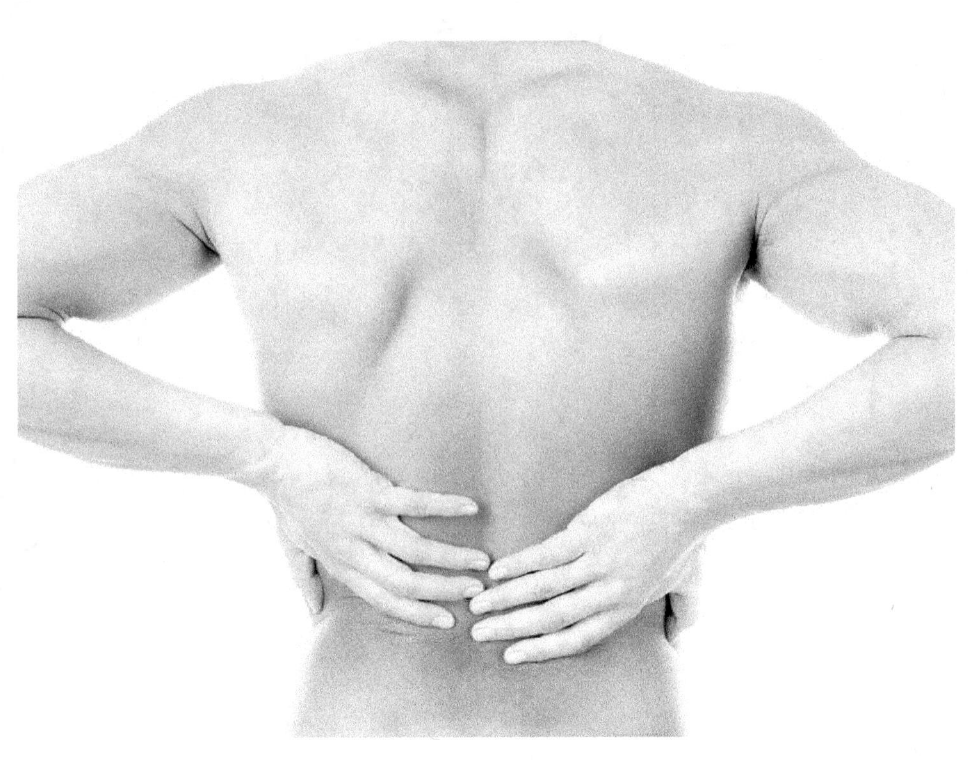